MAKING MICROBLADING FOR BEGINNERS

Practical Knowledge Guide On Skills, Techniques And Pattern To Understand, Master & Explore The Process Of Microblading From Scratch

HENRY HICKMAN

Disclaimer

The information provided in this book has been meticulously researched and compiled to ensure accuracy and completeness. However, it is important to note that the content within this book is intended solely for informational and educational purposes. It is not intended for self-prediction or as a guarantee of outcomes.

The author has dedicated considerable time and effort to present reliable information.

Nevertheless, the author cannot be held responsible for any potential omission of words or content within this book.

Furthermore, the author hereby declares no affiliation or agreement with any website, individual, product or platform in the form of affiliate or any other kind. This book is created purely for educational purposes.

Readers are advised that the author will not be liable for any loss or consequences, whether direct or indirect, arising from the use or misuse of the information contained in this book. It is recommended to exercise discretion and consult additional sources or professionals when implementing the techniques or information provided herein.

By using this book, readers agree to do so at their own discretion and assume full responsibility for any actions taken based on the content presented.

Table of Contents

CHAPTER 1

Introduction

Microblading is a new procedure in the field of beauty and cosmetic treatments that focuses primarily on improving the look of brows. This chapter looks into the complex realm of microblading, investigating its definition, historical antecedents, and the critical function brows play in face aesthetics.

Understanding Microblading

Microblading, commonly referred to as eyebrow embroidery or feathering, is a semi-permanent cosmetic surgery that includes the precise application of pigment to the skin, providing the appearance of larger, well-defined eyebrows. To deposit colors into the skin's surface layers, a manual hand-held instrument with ultra-fine needles is used.

As a consequence, the individual's facial traits are complemented with natural-looking, finely sculpted brows.

In some aspects, microblading differs from regular brow tattooing. Unlike tattoos, which penetrate deeper layers of the skin, microblading is a surface-level method, allowing for a more polished and realistic finish. Furthermore, the manual tool used in microblading allows for higher accuracy, allowing the technician to replicate the look of individual brow hairs.

History And Evolution Of Microblading

Microblading has its origins in ancient civilizations when different types of permanent and semi-permanent cosmetics were employed for aesthetic and cultural objectives. However, the recent comeback of microblading may be ascribed to Asia, where the practice gained popularity in the previous decade.

In recent years, microblading has significantly advanced, with innovations in equipment, pigments, and procedures. This progress has led to the growing acceptance and popularity of microblading as a mainstream cosmetic technique internationally. The combination of traditional craftsmanship and cutting-edge technology has raised microblading to the status of an art form, enabling practitioners to achieve hyper-realistic and individualized outcomes.

Importance Of Eyebrows In Facial Aesthetics

The importance of brows in face beauty cannot be emphasized. Eyebrows define the face, frame the eyes, and contribute to overall facial harmony. Well-shaped brows may improve facial symmetry, give a more youthful look, and bring attention to the eyes.

Understanding the significance of brows in the context of microblading is critical. The process is designed not only to fill in sparse regions or produce a defined form but also to take into account the individual's particular facial characteristics, ensuring that the microbladed brows blend in with the natural curves of the face.

The brows are often used to transmit facial expressions, emotions, and communication. As a result, microblading goes beyond basic cosmetic improvement; it contributes to increased confidence and self-esteem by allowing people to obtain their ideal brow appearance, according to their facial features.

Finally, this introductory chapter gives a basic overview of microblading, tracing its origins from past practices to its modern development. As a background, the relevance of brows in face aesthetics is highlighted, highlighting the necessity of this cosmetic treatment in increasing not only physical look but also psychological well-being. The next chapters will go into the complexities of the microblading technique, aftercare, possible hazards, and the ever-changing environment of this dynamic sector.

CHAPTER 2

Anatomy Of The Eyebrow

Microblading is a delicate skill that includes the precise augmentation of brows using semi-permanent pigment inserted into the epidermis. To master this method, it is necessary to first get a basic grasp of brow anatomy. This chapter delves into the subtle aspects that contribute to the aesthetics and natural beauty of eyebrows, including the structure of eyebrow hair, the eyebrow development cycle, and the different variables that impact eyebrow form.

Structure Of Eyebrow Hair

A microblading artist must first understand the structure of brow hair. Unlike scalp hair, eyebrow hair is finer and shorter. Each hair follicle generates a single brow hair, and the density of these hairs varies from person to person.

The thickness, length, and direction of brow hair all have a role in the overall look of the brows.

The hair follicle, which is located under the skin's surface, is involved in the anatomy of the brow hair. Hair growth is controlled by the hair bulb, which is situated at the base of the follicle. The dermal papilla and matrix surround the hair bulb and perform critical functions in nourishing and maintaining hair development. The sebaceous gland, which is located near the follicle, generates sebum, an oil that aids in the maintenance of hair health and luster.

To make natural-looking hair strokes throughout the technique, microblading artists must understand the complexities of these structures. It is essential to mimic the natural growth pattern and direction of brow hair to get realistic and visually attractive outcomes.

Eyebrow Growth Cycle

The brow hair development cycle is a dynamic process that includes three phases: anagen, catagen, and telogen. Understanding these stages is critical for both microblading artists and customers looking for long-term effects.

Anagen Phase: This is the active growth phase, during which hair root cells divide quickly and new hair is generated. The length of the anagen phase determines the length of the hair.

Catagen Phase: Hair growth slows and the hair follicle shrinks during this transitional phase. This stage is brief, lasting just a few weeks.

Telogen period: The resting period during which old hair is shed and new hair grows. The telogen phase lasts varying amounts of time, and it is at this time that people may shed naturally.

Microblading works best when done during the anagen period when the hair is actively developing and can better maintain the pigmented pigment. Educating customers on the normal growth cycle of brow hair helps in managing expectations about the sustainability of microblading outcomes.

Factors Influencing Eyebrow Shape

Eyebrow form is determined by a mix of genetic, environmental, and personal variables. Microblading artists must take these factors into account to generate unique and pleasing outcomes for each client.

Genetics: An individual's genetic composition plays a crucial part in shaping the natural form and arch of their brows. Microblading enables the improvement of existing characteristics while taking into account the client's genetic predisposition.

Facial Structure: The overall facial structure, which includes the form of the eyes, nose, and forehead, may influence the optimum brow shape. Microblading artists use these characteristics while creating harmonic and balanced brows that suit the client's face.

Personal Preferences: Client preferences and stylistic preferences can have an impact on eyebrow form. Some people want a strong and distinct appearance, while others prefer a softer and more natural appearance. Communication between the microblading artist and the customer is essential for attaining the desired result.

Trends and Fashion: Current trends and fashion influence the ideal brow aesthetics. Microblading artists keep up with changing trends to provide customers with new and stylish options.

Finally, goes into the fine aspects of the anatomy of the eyebrow, such as the formation of eyebrow hair, the development cycle, and the different variables affecting eyebrow shape. A thorough comprehension of these components is essential for every microblading artist who wants to provide great and tailored outcomes for their customers.

CHAPTER 3

Microblading Tools And Equipment

Microblading is a laborious and exact craft that necessitates the use of specialized instruments and equipment. In this chapter, we will look at the fundamental components of the microblading process, such as an overview of the instruments, the many kinds of blades used, and the significance of pigments and color matching.

Overview Of Microblading Tools

1. **Microblading Pen:** A basic instrument used by technicians to make fine, hair-like strokes on the skin is the microblading pen. It is usually made up of a lightweight handle and a blade holding. Different kinds of blades may be added to the blade holder, providing more versatility in stroke patterns.

2. Blade Holder: The microblading pen's blade holder retains the microblading blades. Its purpose is to give stability and control during the operation. The blades are available in a variety of combinations, enabling specialists to tailor the thickness and form of the strokes.

3. Microblading Blades: These tiny, disposable blades are essential for making tiny incisions in the skin where pigment is placed. varied blade shapes, such as U-shaped, slanted, and curved, have varied results. The blade used is determined by criteria such as the desired brow shape and the client's natural brow hair.

4. Measuring instruments: Precision is essential in microblading, and instruments like calipers assist professionals in mapping out the brow form, assuring symmetry and balance.

5. Pigment Rings and Cups: During the treatment, microblading experts utilize tiny rings or cups to contain pigments. To meet sanitary requirements, these containers are often disposable.

6. **Microbrushes and Cotton Swabs:** These are used during and after the treatment to administer anesthesia or to clean and shape the brows.

7. **Skin Marker/Pencil:** Before the treatment, technicians utilize skin markers or pencils to sketch the form of the brows. This acts as a guide for making accurate strokes.

Different Types Of Blades

Microblading blades are crucial in deciding the ultimate result of the treatment. The blade used is determined by parameters such as the client's natural brow hair, skin type, and desired brow shape.

Here are several examples:

1. **U-shaped blades:** Use these blades to create soft, natural-looking brows. They are designed to seem like individual brow hairs.

2. **Slanted Blades:** Slanted blades are often utilized to define and organize the brow contour. They may give the strokes more depth and character.

3. **Curved Blades:** Curved blades are ideal for customers who have a natural brow arch. They are adaptable and may be used to accentuate a variety of brow forms.

Pigments And Color Matching

Choosing the proper pigments and ensuring precise color matching are critical components of microblading. The idea is to produce brows that seem natural and complement the client's skin tone and hair color. Important factors include:

1. **Undertones:** Understanding the client's undertones is critical for choosing the appropriate

pigment. Whether the undertones are warm, cold, or neutral, the pigment should complement the client's entire complexion.

2. Color Mixing: To get the correct shade, microblading experts often combine pigments. This enables personalization depending on the client's distinct qualities and preferences.

3. Patch Testing: A patch test is suggested before the operation to confirm that the selected color does not induce an allergic response. This is an important step in ensuring the client's safety and happiness.

Finally, the tools and equipment utilized in microblading are critical in producing accurate and visually acceptable outcomes. The effectiveness of the microblading technique is dependent on a comprehensive grasp of the different blades, as well as rigorous pigment selection and color matching. The next part of our investigation of microblading will concentrate on the technical process of the microblading procedure itself.

CHAPTER 4

Preparing For Microblading

Microblading, an innovative semi-permanent cosmetic technique, requires thorough planning to get the best outcomes and customer satisfaction. This chapter goes into the critical aspects of microblading preparation, highlighting the importance of client consultation, skin analysis, pre-treatment care, and successfully managing client expectations.

Client Consultation

The cornerstone of a successful microblading operation is a comprehensive client consultation. This first encounter serves many functions, including enabling the technician to learn about the client's preferences, evaluate their expectations, and ensure they are well informed about the procedure.

The technician should address the client's preferred brow shape, thickness, and general aesthetic preferences during the consultation. Analyzing the client's facial traits, such as face shape and eye shape, aids in personalizing the microblading pattern to enhance their natural attractiveness. It's critical to moderate expectations by describing the procedure's limits and clarifying variables that may impact the final result, such as skin type and existing brow hair.

Furthermore, the consultation is an excellent opportunity to learn about the client's medical history, allergies, and any drugs they may be taking. This information is critical for assuring the client's safety and detecting any possible contraindications during the operation.

Skin Analysis And Pre-Treatment Care

A thorough examination of the client's skin is required to establish its eligibility for microblading.

To personalize the technique to the individual, skin type, texture, and any existing disorders must be evaluated. Technicians should be familiar with various skin types and how they affect the healing process and pigment retention.

The importance of pre-treatment care in prepping the skin for microblading cannot be overstated. In the days coming up to the treatment, clients should be encouraged to avoid specific activities and items. To lessen the risk of bleeding during the procedure, avoid alcohol and blood-thinning drugs. Technicians should provide clear instructions on how to prepare the skin, stressing the necessity of having a clean and hydrated surface for the best outcomes.

During this stage, a patch test for pigments may be conducted to determine any possible allergic responses.

This preventative action assures the client's safety and aids in the selection of the best pigments for their skin tone.

Setting Expectations And Managing Client Concerns

Clear communication is critical in managing client expectations and resolving any concerns regarding the microblading procedure. Technicians should describe the probable discomfort of the treatment and the use of numbing drugs to reduce pain. Timelines for the healing process, as well as the predicted duration of the outcomes, should be explained.

It is critical at this time to educate customers on the necessity of aftercare. Providing specific post-treatment care recommendations, such as limiting sun exposure, swimming, and particular skincare products, helps to ensure the effectiveness of the microblading procedure.

Addressing and handling customer concerns is an essential component of the planning process. Technicians should be prepared to answer concerns regarding the procedure's safety, any adverse effects, and the amount of pain to be anticipated. During this phase, developing trust and rapport with customers promotes a good experience and lays the basis for a successful microblading journey.

To summarize, proper preparation for microblading includes a thorough client consultation, a rigorous inspection of the client's skin, and excellent communication to establish realistic expectations. This preparation assures not only the client's safety and comfort but also provides the framework for obtaining visually acceptable and long-lasting outcomes in the fascinating realm of microblading.

CHAPTER 5

Microblading Techniques

Microblading is a cosmetic tattooing method that has grown in popularity due to its ability to produce natural-looking brows. In this chapter, we'll dig into the complicated realm of microblading methods, looking at the creativity behind hair stroke patterns, the differences between feathering and microshading, and how to customize procedures to fit different brow types.

Hair Stroke Patterns

The ability of microblading to resemble the look of natural brow hairs is its defining feature. This requires a thorough grasp of hair stroke patterns. Microblading experts create a smooth and genuine effect by precisely crafting tiny strokes that imitate actual hairs.

In microblading, many hair stroke patterns are used, each having a specific function. The traditional hair stroke pattern entails drawing tiny, precise lines that follow the natural direction of the client's brow hairs. This procedure guarantees that the microbladed brows mix flawlessly with the natural ones, resulting in a natural and harmonious look.

Microblading artists may also experiment with various stroke patterns to generate different results. Diagonal strokes, for example, may add drama, whilst vertical strokes can give a more organized and defined design. The creativity is in selecting the perfect pattern combination to complement the client's facial characteristics and preferences.

Feathering Vs. Microshading

Two basic microblading procedures have developed as popular options: feathering and micro shading.

Understanding the differences between these techniques is essential for microblading artists who want to provide individualized and bespoke solutions to their customers.

Feathering:

The basic microblading method that focuses on making natural-looking hair strokes is feathering, also known as micro feathering or hair stroking. The strokes are carefully carved into the skin, like individual brow hairs. This method is suitable for customers who want a delicate, subtle improvement to their natural brows, resulting in a more discreet but polished look.

Microshading:

Microshading, on the other hand, uses small dots to produce a darkened or powdered look. Clients who like a stronger, more defined appearance often use this approach.

Microshading may give depth and dimension to brows, making them look fuller and more polished. It is especially beneficial for customers who have sparse or uneven brows, as it helps provide a more consistent and filled-in appearance.

Microblading artists often mix feathering and micro-shading methods to provide a personalized outcome that is tailored to the client's specific preferences and face characteristics.

Customizing Techniques For Different Brow Styles

One of the main advantages of microblading is its adaptability to different brow types. Microblading artists must be able to tailor their procedures to each client's specific qualities and preferences.

Architectural Points to Consider:
The architectural structure of the client's face is critical in identifying the best microblading procedure. Bold and defined strokes may be used

to enhance the characteristics of customers with an angular facial shape. A more delicate and feathery technique may be recommended for people with a softer, rounder face.

Color Adjustment:

When personalizing procedures, microblading artists must also consider the client's natural hair color and skin tone. The colors used in microblading should complement the client's current characteristics, resulting in a seamless and natural appearance. This entails choosing the appropriate shade and intensity to get the desired impact.

Adapting to Individual Preferences:

Each customer has different tastes, ranging from a natural, barely-there augmentation to a strong, statement-making style. Microblading artists must actively communicate with their customers to understand their expectations and tailor their skills appropriately. This may include altering the stroke thickness, general contour of the brows, and the degree of shading used.

Finally, perfecting microblading methods is an art form that extends beyond technical ability. It requires a thorough awareness of hair stroke patterns, a sophisticated comprehension of feathering and micro shading differences, and the ability to tailor procedures to various brow designs. Armed with this expertise, microblading artists can produce spectacular and individualized outcomes that complement their customers' inherent attractiveness.

CHAPTER 6

Health And Safety In Microblading

Microblading is a popular cosmetic technique that involves manually implanting pigment into the skin with a small blade to provide semi-permanent brow augmentation. While the outcomes may be life-changing, it is critical to emphasize health and safety throughout the microblading procedure. In this chapter, we will look at the most important aspects of keeping a safe and sanitary environment for both the microblading artist and the customer.

Sterilization And Sanitation

Sterilization:

The complete cleaning of equipment is one of the core cornerstones of health and safety in microblading.

Microblading requires the use of a variety of instruments, such as blades, needles, and pigment cups. To remove the possibility of infection and disease transmission, proper sterilization is required. Autoclaving, a method that sterilizes tools using high-pressure steam, is often used in professional microblading studios.

Sanitation:

In addition to sterilization, a clean and hygienic working environment is essential. All surfaces, including treatment tables, chairs, and worktops, should be cleaned and disinfected regularly. To further decrease the danger of cross-contamination, disposable coverings for surfaces that come into direct touch with customers may be employed.

Infection Prevention

Preparation of the Skin:

It is essential to thoroughly prepare the client's skin before beginning the microblading operation. This entails removing any makeup, oils, or microorganisms from the brow region using a mild, antiseptic solution. A pre-procedure consultation is also necessary to rule out any contraindications or conditions that may raise the risk of infection.

How to Wear Gloves:

Throughout the operation, microblading artists should always use disposable, latex-free gloves. This reduces the possibility of germ spread by preventing direct contact between the artist's hands and the client's skin. Gloves should be replaced between customers, and artists should keep their hands clean.

Infection prevention begins with giving customers clear and precise aftercare instructions. To reduce the risk of infection, clients should be taught how to clean and care for their brows after the treatment. During the first healing time, it is usually best to avoid activities that may expose the treated region to dirt, germs, or excessive wetness.

Safe Handling Of Tools And Pigments

One-Time Use Tools:

Many microblading instruments, including blades and needles, are intended for single use. It is essential to follow this approach and appropriately dispose of these objects after each process.

Reusing instruments raises the potential of cross-contamination and jeopardizes both the client's and the artist's safety.

Containers for Pigment:

To avoid contamination, pigments used in microblading should be distributed into single-use disposable containers. Avoiding direct contact between the pigment container and non-disposable surfaces or instruments should be avoided. Furthermore, any remaining pigment should be removed after the treatment.

Correct Disposal:

Dispose of all disposable objects, including gloves, needles, blades, and pigment containers, in line with local health rules. To avoid needlestick injuries, sharps containers should be used for the proper disposal of blades and needles.

In conclusion, ensuring health and safety in microblading is not only a legal and ethical requirement, but it is also critical to the procedure's effectiveness and the well-being of both the artist and the customer. Strict attention to sterilization and sanitation techniques, infection control measures, and correct tool and pigment handling are critical components in producing a safe and sanitary microblading workplace.

CHAPTER 7

The Microblading Process

Microblading has grown in popularity as a semi-permanent method for creating beautifully defined brows. This chapter will go into the intricacies of the microblading method, from the step-by-step procedure to numbing procedures, pain management, touch-up sessions, and aftercare.

Step-By-Step Procedure

1. Consultation:

Before the microblading operation starts, the customer and the microblading artist have a full consultation. This is an important stage in which the artist discusses the client's expectations and assesses the natural brow form, color, and general face characteristics to design a unique plan.

2. Selecting the Appropriate Shape and Color:

The microblading expert chooses the best brow shape and color for the customer based on their preferences and facial anatomy. This stage requires accuracy as well as an awareness of the client's intended aesthetic output.

3. How to Prepare the Brow Area:

After that, the brow region is carefully cleansed and any existing brow hair is clipped if required. The artist ensures that there are no oils or cosmetics on the skin that might interfere with the microblading procedure.

4. Creating a Brow Outline:
The artist draws the desired brow shape on the client's skin using a specialist pencil or pen. This guideline guides the microblading operation,

ensuring that the end outcome meets the client's expectations.

5. How to Use the Numbing Cream:

A topical numbing lotion is administered to the brow region to reduce pain during the treatment. This cream often includes a mix of lidocaine and prilocaine, which helps decrease discomfort and makes the client's experience more pleasant.

6. Strokes for Microblading:

The microblading artist creates thin, precise strokes that replicate real brow hairs using tiny handheld equipment equipped with sharp needles. The pigment is injected into the skin's surface layers, providing the illusion of bigger, more defined brows.

7. Application of Pigment:

High-quality pigments designed exclusively for microblading are meticulously chosen to match the client's desired hue. The pigment is applied to the microbladed strokes by the artist, assuring uniform dispersion and a unified, natural effect.

8. Symmetry Check:

The artist examines for symmetry and modifies as required during the operation to ensure that both brows are symmetrical and match the client's facial characteristics.

9. Finishing Touches:

Following the completion of the microblading procedure, the artist cleans the treated area and administers a soothing ointment to help in the healing process. Following that, the customer is given aftercare recommendations to ensure the best possible outcomes.

Numbing Techniques And Pain Management

While microblading is typically safe, it might cause some pain. Numbing procedures are critical in ensuring the customer has a pain-free experience. As previously stated, topical numbing creams are widely employed and are used before the microblading treatment. To further reduce any pain, some artists may employ a liquid anesthetic throughout the procedure.

Both the artist and the client must talk honestly about pain tolerances and comfort levels. Some customers may feel just a little pain, however, others may find particular regions to be more sensitive. Because of this connection, the artist can make real-time modifications to provide a good and pain-free microblading experience.

Touch-Up Sessions And Aftercare

Touch-up sessions are an important part of the microblading procedure since it is a semi-permanent solution. These sessions are usually scheduled four to six weeks following the first microblading surgery. The artist examines the healed results, makes any required corrections, and ensures that the color and form stay constant throughout the touch-up session.

Microblading aftercare is critical to its long-term success. To encourage good healing and color retention, clients are urged to follow particular rules. Following-care guidelines often include avoiding excessive wetness, sun exposure, and using specific skincare products on the treated region. Clients are also urged not to scrape or scratch the healing skin to avoid pigment loss.

Finally, microblading is a painstaking craft that requires careful preparation, accuracy, and attention to detail. From the first consultation to the last touch-up session and aftercare, each step adds to the client's overall face aesthetics by producing natural-looking, well-defined brows. As the popularity of microblading grows, the value of professional and experienced microblading artists in producing good results and guaranteeing customer happiness cannot be emphasized.

CHAPTER 8

Common Challenges And Troubleshooting

As a complicated and revolutionary cosmetic treatment, microblading is not without its difficulties. This chapter delves into some of the most typical complications that practitioners may face during microblading sessions, as well as helpful troubleshooting procedures.

Dealing With Uneven Pigmentation

One of the most difficult aspects of microblading is attaining uniform and even pigmentation. unequal pigmentation may be caused by a variety of circumstances, including unequal pressure application, variable needle depth, or differences in the client's skin type. Addressing this problem demands a methodical approach.

Technique Refinement: To maintain consistent pigmentation, practitioners should constantly enhance their microblading procedures. Consistent pressure and controlled strokes are required for even outcomes. Regular training and skill development may greatly aid in mastering this technique.

Correct Needle Selection: The selection of needles is critical in pigmentation. Using the correct needle for the skin type and the desired goal might assist in reducing uneven pigmentation. Fine needles are appropriate for sensitive regions, while bigger needles may be required for stronger strokes.

Touch-Up Sessions: Offering touch-up sessions to rectify uneven pigmentation is a regular practice. These sessions enable practitioners to fine-tune the color and achieve a more balanced look. It is critical to communicate with customers about the potential of touch-ups and their usefulness in getting ideal outcomes.

Addressing Allergic Reactions

While most people are not sensitive to the pigments used in microblading, allergic reactions may occur. Recognizing and regulating these emotions is critical for the practitioner's and client's health.

Patch Testing: Before the whole treatment, a patch test is required to detect any allergies. This entails applying a small quantity of pigment to a discrete region of the client's skin and monitoring for any unwanted effects. This preventative strategy may help to avoid serious allergic reactions during the surgery.

Using Hypoallergenic Products: Using hypoallergenic colors and numbing lotions may reduce the likelihood of allergic responses.

These products are designed to be softer on the skin, lowering the possibility of unwanted reactions. Thorough investigation and selection of trustworthy, high-quality items are critical.

Emergency Planning: Despite precautions, allergic responses may occur. Practitioners should be prepared to deal with situations as soon as they arise. Having an emergency bag stocked with antihistamines and other necessary drugs might help to mitigate severe responses.

Correcting Shape And Symmetry Issues

Achieving the right shape and symmetry in microblading is an art form, yet obstacles may occur while aiming for perfection. Uneven brows, asymmetry, and unhappiness with the final form are all common problems.

Extensive discussions: It is important to conduct extensive discussions with customers to understand their expectations and preferences. Clear communication regarding the procedure's limits and the inherent differences in brow structure may help manage expectations and reduce unhappiness.

Skill improvement: Addressing form and symmetry concerns requires ongoing skill improvement. Practitioners should devote time to continued training to hone their creative ability and keep current on the newest microblading trends and methods.

Corrective procedures: When form and symmetry problems persist, corrective procedures may be used. This might include further microblading strokes to shape the form or the usage of pigment removal methods. Correction, on the other hand, should be handled with care to prevent overworking the skin.

To summarize, managing the hurdles of microblading requires a mix of technical competence, artistic elegance, and a dedication to continuous learning. Practitioners may improve their customers' overall pleasure and safety by addressing uneven pigmentation, allergic responses, and form and symmetry difficulties with precision and care.

CHAPTER 9

Marketing And Building Your Microblading Business

Effective marketing methods and a solid internet presence are critical components for the success of a microblading company in the ever-changing beauty industry scene. This chapter goes into the complexities of marketing methods, the significance of having a strong web presence, customer retention strategies, and legal and licensing issues for microblading practitioners.

Client Retention Strategies

Building a loyal clientele is critical to the long-term viability of a microblading firm. Client retention techniques include providing a great experience, staying in touch, and promoting repeat business.

1. Outstanding Customer Service:

- Deliver an amazing customer experience from the minute they ask about your services until their microblading process is completed. Make them feel respected and at ease throughout the process.

- Follow up with customers after their appointments to guarantee their satisfaction and to resolve any problems as soon as possible.

2. Client Loyalty Programs:

- Create loyalty programs to reward repeat customers. Provide discounts or free services to customers who recommend people to your company.

- Send out newsletters or emails to your customers regularly to keep them up to date on specials, new services, and industry developments.

3. Reliable Communication:

- Maintain constant and open contact with your clientele. During significant events, send appointment reminders, follow-up notes, and customized greetings.

- Seek feedback actively and utilize it to enhance your services. You may enhance your connection with your clientele by demonstrating that you appreciate their views.

Legal And Licensing Considerations

To maintain compliance with health and safety regulations, running a microblading company requires adhering to legal and regulatory procedures.

1. Certification and Licensing:

- Research and adhere to your jurisdiction's licensing regulations for microblading practitioners. Obtain the qualifications required to show your proficiency in the industry.

- Stay up to speed on any modifications or changes to licensing laws to prevent legal snafus.

2. Compliance with Health and Safety Regulations:

- To safeguard both clients and practitioners, certain health and safety regulations must be implemented. Follow sanitation rules, utilize disposable instruments when appropriate, and keep your workstation clean and sanitary.

3. Insurance Protection:
- Obtain insurance for your microblading company. This may include professional liability insurance to safeguard your studio from any legal claims as well as property insurance.

4. Consent of the Client and Documentation:

- Create detailed client permission documents that outline the risks and advantages of microblading. Ascertain that the operation, aftercare instructions, and possible results are understood by the customers.

- Maintain meticulous records of each client's consultation, procedure, and any negative responses. In the event of a legal issue, proper documentation might be critical.

Finally, good marketing, customer retention, and legal concerns are critical components of establishing and maintaining a prosperous microblading company. Microblading specialists may develop a respected and long-lasting presence in the beauty market by creating a strong web presence, executing successful client retention techniques, and complying with regulatory and licensing regulations.

CHAPTER 10

Advancements In Microblading

Microblading, a cutting-edge procedure in the field of permanent cosmetics, has made considerable strides in recent years. This chapter goes into the most recent developments, cutting-edge technology, and the significance of continuous education in the ever-changing area of microblading.

Emerging Trends In Eyebrow Enhancement

1. **Natural-looking outcomes**: Pursuing natural-looking outcomes is a popular trend in microblading. Clients are increasingly preferring brows that complement their facial characteristics without seeming too manipulated. Skilled microblading artists use procedures that mirror

the appearance of natural hair, resulting in a delicate and realistic effect.

2. **Ombré Brows:** In recent years, ombré brows, which have a progressive transition from a lighter to a darker hue, have gained popularity. This method creates a delicate and defined appearance, providing customers with a contemporary alternative to classic solid-fill brows.

3. **Feathered Brows:** Feathered brows, also called fluffy or soap brows, entail making your brows seem wispy and feathery. This style mimics the natural growth pattern of brow hair, resulting in a delicate and ethereal appearance that is in high demand.

4. On the opposite end of the scale, some customers like strong and graphic brows. Microblading specialists create statement brows

that stand out with precise strokes and clever shading.

New Technologies And Tools

1. Digital Mapping and Design: As technology advances, digital mapping and design tools have entered the domain of microblading. Artists may now employ specialized software to generate exact templates and designs that are suited to each client's particular face shape, resulting in a more accurate and individualized result.

2. The development of high-quality pigments and excellent color-matching technology has changed the microblading business. Artists are now able to create a larger variety of hues, allowing for more personalization to match the client's real hair color and skin tone.

3. Automated Microblading Equipment: With the emergence of automated equipment, traditional handheld microblading instruments have experienced innovation. These equipment often have variable needle speeds and precise control mechanisms, which improve the overall accuracy and efficiency of the microblading procedure.

Continuing Education In Microblading

1. Evolving Techniques and Trends: Because the beauty business is ever-changing, microblading artists understand the need to remain up to date on new techniques and trends. Continuous learning via workshops, seminars, and online courses guarantees that artists can provide the most up-to-date and in-demand services to their clientele.

2. Protocols for Safety and Hygiene: As with any cosmetic treatment, keeping high standards of safety and hygiene is critical in microblading. Ongoing education stresses current procedures, sterilizing methods, and best practices to protect the artist's and client's safety.

3. Client Communication and Consulting Skills: In addition to technical knowledge, continuing education in microblading often involves instruction in efficient client communication and consulting. This is critical for recognizing and satisfying each customer's expectations and preferences, creating healthy connections, and ensuring client satisfaction.

Finally, the discipline of microblading is evolving as a result of developing trends, technical improvements, and a dedication to continued education. Microblading artists who embrace these innovations are better positioned to produce great, tailored outcomes that reflect their clients' various tastes.

Conclusion

Recap Of Key Takeaways

In conclusion, microblading is a precise and creative technique that requires talent, accuracy, and a thorough grasp of particular client requirements. A microblading artist's success is determined by their ability to produce natural-looking, tailored brows while emphasizing client safety and happiness. Training and certification are critical in developing essential skills and establishing a reputation in the field.

Encouragement For Aspiring Microblading Artists

Continuous study and practice are essential for individuals wishing to join the field of microblading. Accept obstacles as chances to improve your skill, and seek advice from seasoned specialists. A successful career in microblading requires a mix of technical skill, creative flare, and a dedication to providing extraordinary outcomes.

Looking Towards The Future Of Microblading

Artists should be versatile and open to embracing new methods and technology as the field of microblading grows. With prospective breakthroughs in pigments, equipment, and processes, the future presents intriguing possibilities. The key to success in the microblading business is a dedication to quality, ethical procedures, and a desire to enhance customers' inherent attractiveness via this transforming art form.

In conclusion, microblading is more than just a cosmetic procedure; it is an art form that allows people to feel confident and attractive.

Microblading artists may carve out a fulfilling and long-lasting career in this dynamic and changing area by embracing continual development, remaining current on industry trends, and emphasizing client happiness.

THE END